ALL YOU

Knee Joint
Pain

Edited by
Dr Savitri Ramaiah

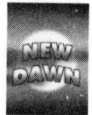

New Dawn

NEW DAWN PRESS GROUP

Published by New Dawn Press Group
New Dawn Press, Inc., 244 South Randall Rd # 90, Elgin, IL 60123
e-mail: sales@newdawnpress.com

New Dawn Press, 2 Tintern Close, Slough, Berkshire, SL1-2TB, UK
e-mail: sterlingdis@yahoo.co.uk

New Dawn Press (An Imprint of Sterling Publishers (P) Ltd.)
A-59, Okhla Industrial Area, Phase-II, New Delhi-110020
e-mail: sterlingpublishers@airtelmail.in
www.sterlingpublishers.com

All You Wanted to Know About - Knee Joint Pain
© 1999, Sterling Publishers Private Limited
ISBN 978-81-207-2229-3
Reprint 2002, 2007, 2009

PRINTED IN INDIA

Information for this series, has been provided by *Health Update*, a monthly bulletin of the Society for Health Education and Learning Packages. The Update is intended to provide you with knowledge to adopt preventive measures and cooperate with the doctor during illness for better outcome of treatment.

Contributors

ALLOPATHY
Dr. J. Maheswari
(Assistant Professor, Department of Orthopedics, AIIMS, New Delhi)

ACUPUNCTURE
Dr. Ratnakant Patil
(Consultant, Acupuncture, Bangalore)

AYURVEDA
Dr. V.N. Pandey
(Former Director, Central Council for Research in Ayurveda and Siddha, New Delhi)

HOMOEOPATHY
Dr. Sangeeta Chopra
(Consultant Homoeopathy, New Delhi)

NATURE CURE
Dr. Sambhashiva Rao
(Former Chief Medical Officer, Institute of Naturopathy, Bangalore)

UNANI
Hakim Mohammed Khalid Siddiqui
(Director, Central Council for Research in Unani, New Delhi)

Preface

All You Wanted to Know About is an easy-to-read reference series put together by *Health Update* and assisted by a team of medical experts who offer the latest perspectives on body health.

Each book in the series enhances your knowledge on a particular health issue. It makes you an active participant by giving multiple perspectives to choose from — allopathy, acupuncture, ayurveda, homoeopathy, nature cure and unani.

This book is intended as a home adviser but does not substitute a doctor.

The opinions are those of the contributors, and the publisher holds no responsibility.

Contents

Introduction

Most common joint pain is in the knee joint. This can be caused due to two reasons — the special design of the knee joint which makes it relatively unstable secondly they bear the burden of the whole body at every step.

Pain in the knee joint could be due to an injury to the knee, a tear or a facture arthritis. Arthritis is not a disease but a symptom that something is wrong in the joint.

All forms of medicine prefer precautionary measure rather than a cure. Exercises are recommended to maintain normal health.

ALLOPATHY

Joint pain is not only unpleasant but also causes a lot of anxiety. The inability to carry out normal movements efficiently and the fear of being crippled often cause a lot of anxiety. Joint pain can be due to several causes and the treatment varies depending upon the cause of the pain. In recent times, several new developments in the management of joint pains have led to improved treatment of several common causes of joint pain.

Joint pain is a common complaint. It is often associated with aging process. However, it can also occur in children, young adults and middle-aged people. Of the joint pains, pain in the knee joint is the most common. This is because of two main reasons:

• the special design of the knee joint which makes it relatively unstable; and

• the fact that the body-weight passes through the knee joint every time you take a step. It is a great advantage to have a joint in the middle of the length of the leg.

Imagine how it would be without the knee! You would then walk on two pegs, wouldn't be able to sit on the floor, squat or sit cross-legged.

What is the design of the knee joint?

The knee joint consists of:

- bones;

- a *capsule* which covers the joint;

- *synovial fluid* which lubricates the joint;

- *ligaments,* which prevent abnormal movement;

- muscles, which hold the joint together; and

- *menisci* which are sickle shaped and act like cushions of the joint.

Fig 1. Bones of the Knee Joint

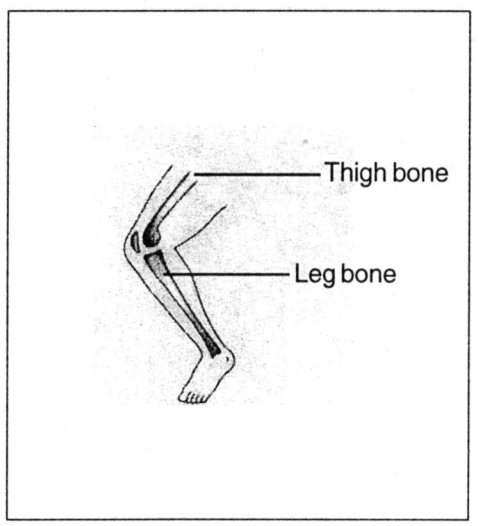

Each of these parts of the knee joint is described below so that you can understand the knee joint better.

Bones. The knee joint, like any other joint, is a junction of two bones:

- the thigh-bone and

- the leg-bone, as shown in Figure 1. The broad ends of these two bones connect with each other in such a way that they can glide over each other. The knee joint is almost like a "hinge" between the two halves of a suitcase. A small bone commonly called the "knee cap" covers the front of the knee. It is fixed firmly in the thigh-muscle and connects with the front of the lower-end of the thigh bone (Figure 2.)

Capsule. The connecting ends of the thigh and leg bones are enclosed in a sheet of cloth-like tissue called the *capsule*. The connecting surfaces of these two bones are covered with the *articular cartilage*. This cartilage is a glistening-white, smooth-like-a-marble, layer. The extraordinary smoothness of the articular cartilage prevents wearing off of

Fig 2. Knee Cap

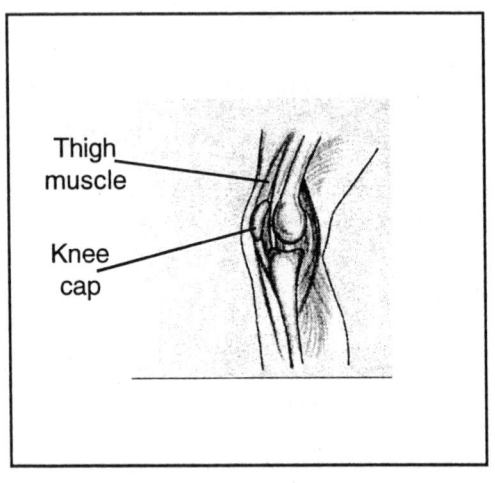

Thigh
muscle

Knee
cap

the connecting joint surfaces when they glide against each other.

Synovial fluid. The lubrication fluid inside the human joints is called the *synovial fluid*. This fluid works like oil in a machine. The "rubbing force" or the force of friction which spoils all moving machines over a period of time is minimum in the joint because of the synovial fluid.

Ligaments. Strap like tissues which join two bones are called the *ligaments*. The knee joint which is designed for movement gets extraordinary strength from these

Fig 3. Ligaments of the Knee Joint

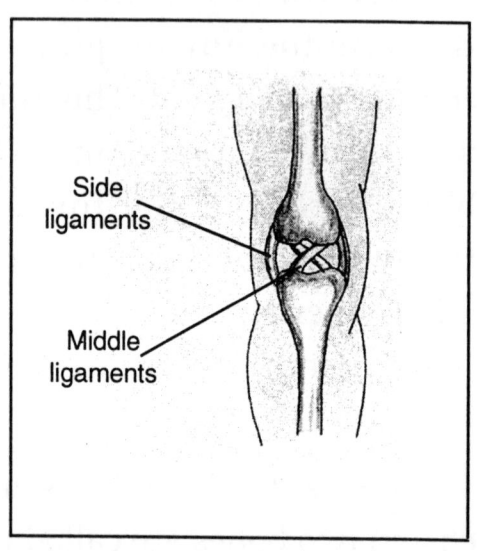

Side ligaments

Middle ligaments

ligaments. Have you ever wondered why the "knee-hinge" does not buckle under the load of

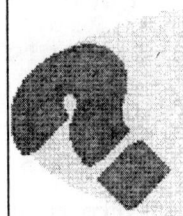

DID YOU KNOW THAT
The knee cap is the largest sesamoid bone of the body. Sesamoid bones are bones which are enbedded in tendon, (the glistening tissue that attaches muscle to the bomne).

your weight while standing? Or how does it hold despite the tremendous force across it when you jump or run? It is because the ligaments act as checks against any load on the joint which tries to force it open on any one side.

There are four main ligaments of the knee — two on the sides and two in the middle as shown in Figure 3. The two side ligaments prevent side-to-side opening of the joint. The two middle ligaments, which are arranged in the form of a cross, prevent abnormal forward and backward movement. Of the two middle ligaments, the front ligament is most commonly ruptured in knee injuries.

Muscles. The muscles around the knee also play a very important role in providing stability to the knee. There are two groups of muscles which control the knee:

• muscles in the front of the thigh, called *quadriceps*; and

• muscles at the back, called *hamstrings*. These muscles contract powerfully and hold the joint in one position in movements such as jumping. The muscles stabilize the joint just as ropes stabilize the pole of a tent.

Menisci. Menisci are made of rubber like tough tissue called cartilage. They are half-moon shaped and are therefore popularly

Fig 4. Semi-lunar Cartilages in the Knee Joint

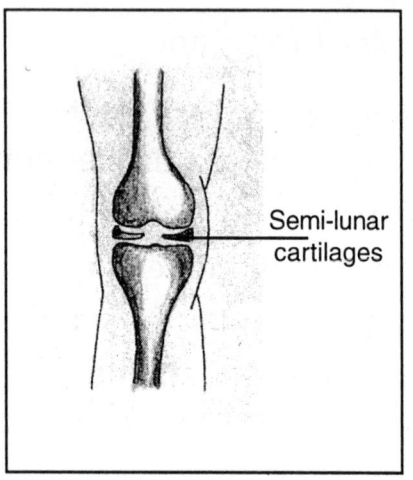

Semi-lunar cartilages

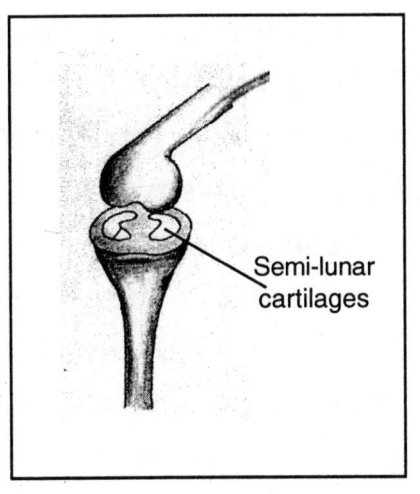

Semi-lunar
cartilages

known as semilunar cartilage. There are two semilunar cartilages in each knee — one on the inner-side and one on the outer-side (Figure 4). The menisci, like washers in a joint, act as space-fillers. They also participate in weight-transmission across the knee. These cartilages can tear if they are caught between the connecting surfaces of the bone. A torn meniscus is an important cause of pain in the knee, particularly in younger, physically active persons. Cricket and football players often suffer from torn menisci.

What are the causes of knee pain?

Knee pain may subside on its own within a few days or persist for weeks or months. When the pain subsides within a few days, it is often due to minor problems such as a 'sprain'. When the knee pain persists for longer time, its causes can:

1. Pain due to injury to the knee;
2. Pain due to conditions not associated with injury.

Knee Sprain — causes and symptoms

• Common in day-to-day activities due to minor twisting or bending.

• Pain subsides within a few days to a week.

• Injury to semilunar cartilages.

• Caused when the knee is twisted or while landing on the knee suddenly.

• Pain may not subside within a few days.

• May give a feeling of something "getting stuck" or "loose" inside the knee.

• Knee may be locked in one position.

Injury to ligaments of the knee — causes and symptoms

• Front middle ligament often injured in sports when a sudden load comes on the knee or while jumping from a height.

• May also be due to forced twisting of the knee.

• May result in a 'sound' of something breaking inside the knee when the ligaments are injured.

• Rapid swelling of the knee because the blood fills the joint.

Fractures and dislocations — causes and symptoms

Fractures may involve

• lower end of the thigh bone,

• upper end of the bone or

• the kneecap.

• Acute pain with immediate swelling.

• Knee cap dislocation is common in adolescents.

• Recurrent dislocation of knee cap is common.

Overuse injuries — causes and symptoms

• Common in sports persons and military recruits due to excessive demand on the joint.

• Pain occurs when adolescents or fresh military recruits undertake new or excessive physical activity.

• Injuries are usually due to a mild problem in the 'design' of the knee.

• Overuse injuries usually cause pain under stressful situation.

Injury to the knee is common in sports, accidents and sometimes day-to-day activities. It is a common cause of knee pain in younger people. There are several types of injuries to the knee joint such as tears in the meniscus, ligaments, etc. which are collectively known as 'Internal Derangement of the Knee' (or 'I.D.K'). Sometimes it is difficult to diagnose the exact type of derangement, and therefore some people consider I.D.K. as synonymous with 'I Don't Know'.

Some causes of knee pain are not associated with injury and often cause pain in other joints also. The main group of diseases in this category is *arthritis*. *The word "arthritis" does not mean one disease — it means pain and swelling of a joint.* There could be many reasons for this type of pain and swelling in the joint. *It is important to remember that different types of arthritis occur at different ages and each one of them has a different outcome. Do not therefore worry unnecessarily if your doctor says that you have arthritis.*

What are the types of knee injury?

Injury to the knee joint is quite common. As mentioned earlier, this is because the design of the knee makes it relatively unstable. It is also prone to injuries because of the stress the knee is subjected to. Causes and symptoms of common knee injuries have been listed before. Described below are the management options for these injuries.

• *Knee sprain.* Minor twisting or bending of the knee result in a sprain which indicates that some tissues around the knee are pulled. Since pain due to sprain subsides within a few days to a week, *you should consult a doctor immediately if the pain persists for more than three weeks, or if the swelling around the knee increases steadily.* Your doctor may recommend rest in a plaster cast or crepe bandage for a few weeks.

• *Injury to semilunar cartilages.* The inner half-moon shaped or semilunar cartilage is more likely to be injured than the outer cartilage. Although cartilage injuries may seem insignificant, they can cause considerable damage to the structures inside the knee. Your doctor may suspect a cartilage tear if the pain does not subside in a few days. If the knee gets 'locked' in one position consult a doctor immediately to free it by manual manipulation.

Most injuries to the knee can cause repeated complaints. It is often difficult to pinpoint the exact nature of the damage by knowing the history of the injury and examination of the knee joint. Your doctor may then suggest a procedure called *"arthroscopy"* in which the doctor looks directly into the joint through a thin pencil like tube called the *arthroscope*. The arthroscope is introduced into the knee through a small cut in the skin. A video-camera is attached to the arthroscope, which shows the inside of the knee on a television. Through this procedure, your doctor will be able to view all the corners of the joint and may therefore be able to identify the cause of symptoms and nature of damage. In most cases, the fault within the joint can be corrected by "key-hole surgery" with the help of small instruments inserted through a few more small cuts. This often avoids a major operation, enables quick recovery and reduces hospital stay to less than forty-eight hours. Arthroscopy not only helps in diagnosing a problem that was not diagnosed earlier but also provides a method of performing surgery with minimum cutting. This technique is therefore a boon for patients with joint problems. However, presently arthroscopy facility is available only at few centres in India.

• *Injury to ligaments of the knee.*
Minor ligament tear such as sprain
may heal on its own. If the tear in
the ligament is complete or more
than one ligament is torn at a time,
the knee may not regain its normal
strength. You may feel unstable
from the day of the injury itself. If
the front middle ligament alone is
torn, there may not be any
symptoms soon after the injury.
After a period of time, you may feel
'weak' on the injured side and knee
pain may develop. Most people
with torn ligaments feel better with
regular special exercises and

careful movements of the knee in day to day activities. However, if the weakness persists, your doctor may recommend a major operation to replace the torn ligament with a new ligament constructed from other body tissues.

• *Fractures and dislocations.* X-rays of the knee are necessary to diagnose the extent of bone(s) damage due to the fracture. In most cases a major operation is necessary to fix the fractured pieces to their normal position with screws and steel plates. These steel plates result in normal movement at the knee. The pain and swelling subsides over a period of time.

• *Overuse injuries.* Knee injuries due to new or excessive physical activity is usually because of a mild problem in the 'design' of the knee. This problem may not routinely cause pain but can do so under stressful situations. It may not be necessary to give up physical activity that has resulted in knee pain. instead, you should undertake strenuous physical activities only after receiving appropriate training and avoid excessive physical stress.

Arthritis

Arthritis is not a disease but a symptom which indicates that "something" is wrong in a joint. Arthritis occurs at all ages but is more common in the elderly. It is least serious among the elderly while it can be serious, crippling and sometimes even life-threatening in young women and children. Of the various types of arthritis, osteoarthritis and rheumatoid arthritis are the most common.

What is osteoarthritis?

Osteoarthritis is destruction of the smooth cartilage covering the ends of the bones. This destruction is similar to the wear and tear of moving machines. It usually starts in the middle age without any specific cause. You may have seen elderly persons walking like a duck, or using a stick to walk. Most of these people suffer from osteoarthritis.

What are the stages of osteoarthritis of the Knee?

In **early stages** there is pain or catch in the knee while

• getting up from siting position or

• changing position of the knee after a period of rest in one position.

In an **later stages**, pain is almost constant and becomes worse on exertion. At this stage the pain is relieved by

- rest;
- pain killer medicines; or
- oil massage.

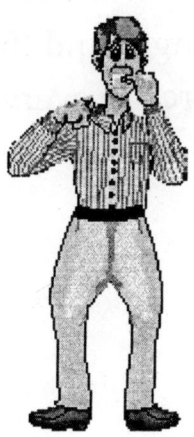

In **advanced stage**, walking is difficult and often needs a lot of effort. Going up and down the stairs is especially very difficult.

The knee may appear 'swollen' and thigh may appear thin. The shape of the legs changes and the knee bows outwards. At this stage, the gait changes and there may be sideways lurch at every step.

What are the causes of osteoarthritis?

Common causes of osteoarthritis are:

• Wear-and-tear due to prolonged use of the joint (This is the commonest cause of osteoarthritis);

• Defect in quality of the cartilage such as in a disease called *pseudogout*;

• Defect in alignment of the articulating surfaces;

- Loose structures inside the joint such as a loose cover of the meniscus;

- Old injury; and

- Previous infection.

What are the risk groups for osteoarthritis?

Osteoarthritis may run in families. It is more common in obese people and those who use the knee excessively such as for sports, standing for a long time or working for long hours with knee in extreme positions. Osteoarthritis is 10 time more common in females than in the males. People with bowed legs develop osteoarthritis much earlier.

What are the symptoms of osteoarthritis of the knee?

Osteoarthritis of the knee is more common among people above fifty years of age, especially the obese. Most people with osteoarthritis complain of pain and/or creaking sound in the knee.

Many people who believe that knee pain means beginning of old age do not always consult with a doctor. It is important to remember that knee pain can occur at all ages and some causes are curable. Also, there are some diseases which may start as a mild pain but rapidly progress to destroy the knee joint.

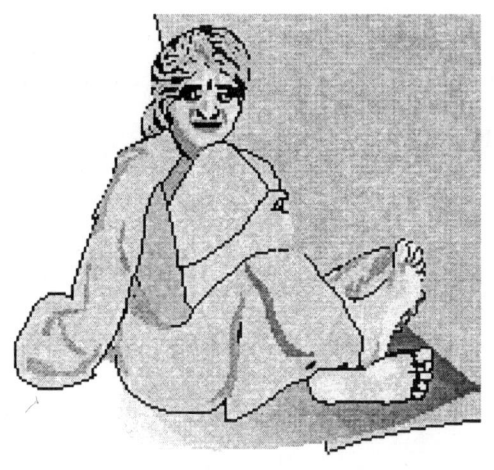

Early diagnosis and timely management that can prevent the progress of an otherwise progressive disease.

When to consult with a doctor?

You should consult with a doctor, especially orthopedic surgeon if you have:

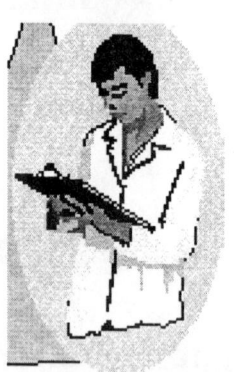

• Pain or stiffness in one joint only or if one joint is affected more than the other;

- Repeated swelling of the knee with pain;

- Symptoms suggestive of a mechanical fault as sudden clicking, something either moving or loose inside the joint.

- Recent bowing of the legs with pain or the inner side of the knee.

- Walking about within the house is difficult due to pain.

What is the management of osteoarthritis?

Osteoarthritis is not curable. Once it starts, it remains for rest of the life. However, *you can relieve the symptoms and minimise disability with timely treatment.* Management of osteoarthritis is through

• non-surgical methods in early stages and

• surgical methods in advanced stages.

What is the non-surgical management of osteoarthritis?

The patient has to do the following for non-surgical management of osteoarth rites.

Patient education. You may start worrying about being crippled 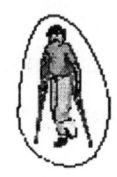 because of arthritis. Your doctor will, therefore, give you a very true picture of your condition which will help lessen your fears and anxiety.

Weight reduction. Regular and adequate exercise may be a 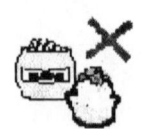 problem if you have difficulty in walking. You may, however, do cycling or swimming regularly. It is, therefore, important to modify your diet and avoid high calorie foods such as sugar, sweets, rice, potato, oil or ghee.

Avoid the following which put excessive stress on the knee:

• Sitting on the floor, in low chairs, sofa or beds.

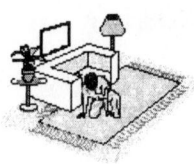 • Squatting, sitting cross-legged and using Indian style toilets.

• Exercises in which you have stand or walk for a long time.

You may get relief by:

• Doing exercises where you can sit on a chair or stool.

• Doing specific exercises to build up the muscles around the knee for providing support to the 'weak' knee.

• Occasional use of medicines to relieve pain. Paracetamol is a safer medicine.

What is the surgical management of osteoarthritis?

Three types of surgeries are recommended for management of osteoarthritis. These include:

- arthroscopy;

- correction of the alignment of the knee; and

- changing the knee joint. None of these surgeries cure osteoarthritis. Your doctor may recommend anyone of these options depending upon the condition of your knee.

- **Arthroscopy.** Your doctor may recommend if you either have

- mechanical problems such as something stuck or loose inside the joint or

- repeated swelling of the knee joint. Although the relief may be partial or temporary, it is often recommended because it is a safe and 'minor' procedure.

As mentioned earlier, your doctor can view the inside of the knee directly through an arthroscope and assess the condition of the cartilage covering

Fig. 6 Alignment of the knee

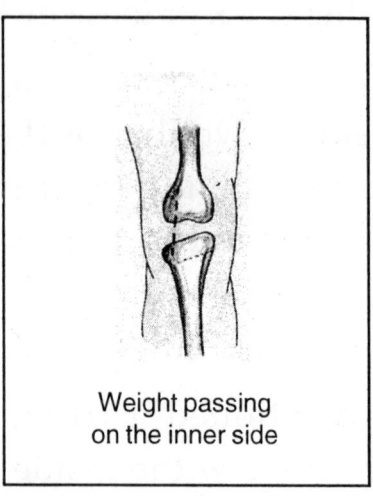

Weight passing
on the inner side

(a)

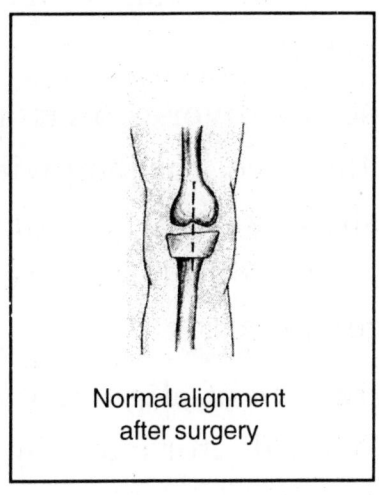

Normal alignment
after surgery

(b)

the bone-ends and the semi-lunar cartilages. Your doctor will also be able to remove (a) any loose or torn pieces of semi-lunar or articular cartilages or

• loose or over-grown tissue lining the knee. The joint will then be washed thoroughly with saline water to completely remove damaged pieces.

• **Correction of alignment of the knee.** Your doctor may suggest a surgery called *High tibial osteotomy* (HTO) to correct the alignment of the knee. This surgery is usually recommended if you have painful osteoarthritis of the knee with bowing of the legs. When your legs are bowed, more body weight passes through the inner side than the outer side of the knee. During the surgery the bone just below the knee is cut and realigned so that the more body weight passes through the outer side of the knee. (Figure 6) After this surgery more than seventy percent patients have relief from pain for almost eight to ten years. It is effective for mild to moderate arthritis, and people who are either young or not obese.

High tibial osteotomy or HTO is a major surgery and requires a

Fig. 7 Changing the knee joint

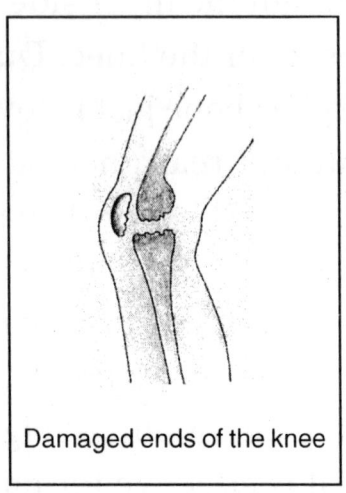

Damaged ends of the knee

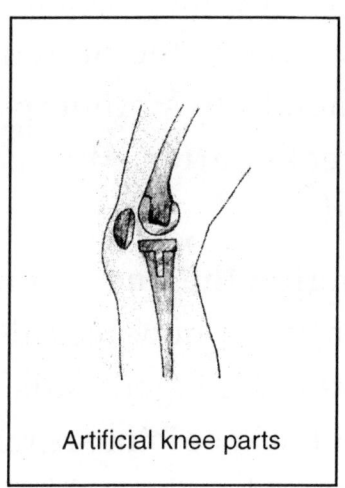

Artificial knee parts

plaster cast for a month after the operation. You can however start walking to the toilet with the plaster about one week after the surgery. Your doctor will also recommend physiotherapy for a few weeks after the cast is removed.

• **Changing the knee joint.** This is a relatively new technique in which the damaged ends of the bones of the knee joint are removed and replaced with artificial parts. A cup-like part is fixed on the end of the thigh bone and a plate-like part is fixed on the end of the leg bone with a special glue called bone-cement (Figure 7). The new parts of the knee are smooth and therefore there is not pain during normal movements of the joint. Although this surgery gives instant relief from pain, it is not always effective. You may have to observe several restrictions in movements so that the new joint may last long. The new joint may last for five to eight years. Also, the artificial knee joint is very expensive and may cost about Rupees sixty thousand. This surgery is usually recommended for people who are not able to walk within the house also.

Rheumatoid Arthritis

What is rheumatoid arthritis?

Rheumatoid arthritis is a disease in which the body develops 'allergy' to some components of the blood. These components accumulate in the joints and some other parts of the body. The body's natural defence mechanism reacts adversely to this accumulation. The result is swelling and pain. Rheumatoid arthritis can cripple a person rapidly, is often extensive and may sometimes even be life-threatening. It is more common in women twenty to forty years of age and may run in families.

What are the symptoms of rheumatoid arthritis?

Early symptoms of rheumatoid arthritis are fever with vague aches and pains in the body including the joints. After about four to six weeks the symptoms are more severe and the pain is present in several joints, especially the joints of the hands and feet. Knee is a major joint and is therefore usually affected. Walking may become difficult. If you do not walk enough, your thigh muscles may become wasted or thin. Rheumatoid arthritis may affect various systems of the body such as the eyes, lungs and the heart. Severity of the symptoms of rheumatoid arthritis is not constant. The symptoms may completely disappear and appear again after some time.

You should consult with a doctor as soon as possible if you have pain and swelling one or more joints. *It is important to remember that all joint pains and swelling are not due to rheumatoid arthritis.*

What is the difference between osteoarthritis and rheumatoid arthritis?

Osteoarthritis usually begins after the age of forty years over a period of several years. It usually begins on joints on one side of the body. It usually affects joints in the knee, hips, hands, feet and the backbone. There are no associated symptoms such as fatigue, fever or loss of weight.

Rheumatoid arthritis starts between twenty five to forty years of age and the symptoms may appear and disappear without any warning. It affects joints on both sides of the body at the same time. It affects most joints including knuckles, wrist and elbows. Rheumatoid arthritis is usually accompanied with fever, weight loss and fatigue.

What is the laboratory test for rheumatoid arthritis?

Your doctor may recommend a test called the R.A. factor. Although this test often helps in diagnosis, it is not always reliable. This is because it is occasionally positive in people who do not have rheumatoid arthritis. Your doctor will therefore diagnose your condition on the basis of history, physical examination and laboratory tests.

What is the management of rheumatoid arthritis?

The basic principles for management of rheumatoid arthritis and other associated diseases. These include:

• *Correct diagnosis.* Since rheumatoid arthritis is just one type of arthritis which involves multiple joints, it is important for you to consult with a doctor, especially a joint-disease specialist (Rheumatologist) and trust his/her judgment. Your doctor may not be able to make the diagnosis before six weeks.

• *Patient education.* Since rheumatoid arthritis is potentially crippling, it is important for you to avoid anxiety. Your doctor will give you details about the course of the disease such as its fluctuating course, long-term treatment options, need to use more than one medicines which may have several adverse impacts, cost of treatment and the need to consult the doctor regularly. You can limit the adverse impacts of the disease by following your doctors recommendations.

• *Avoid treatment from doctors who are not qualified.* Several self-styled doctors may promise your magic cure for rheumatoid arthritis. It is however important to remember that although some medicines may be partially effective for other types of arthritis, rheumatoid arthritis requires a well-planned management schedule.

• *Avoid steroids.* Steroids are chemical substances produced by some glands in the body. They are also available as medicines. Although steroids may give immediate relief you will require larger and larger dose to relieve symptoms over a period of time. They have serious side-effects on almost all parts of the body. Of these, weight-gain, swelling of the face, excess hair growth on the face, reduced vision due to cataract, ulcers and weakness of bones are more common.

• *Diet.* Rheumatoid arthritis does not require any special diet. Avoiding some food items are not likely to cure the disease. You may however have loss of appetite and anaemia. You should therefore eat a balanced diet preferably as small and frequent meals.

• *Moderate activity.* Bed rest is not necessary, except in early 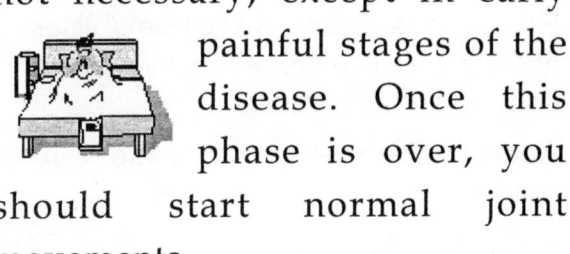 painful stages of the disease. Once this phase is over, you should start normal joint movements.

• *Physiotherapy.* It is very important to start physiotherapy after the disease is controlled a little by medicines. Physiotherapy helps to regain joint mobility and strength. You can do the recommended exercises and heat

Box 1. Principle of management of rheumatoid arthritis

Correct diagnosis, preferably by a Rheumatologist.

Education regarding the course of illness and adverse effects of the disease and its management options.

Acceptance that the disease is not curable.

Avoid steroids.

Eat small frequent balanced meals.

Do simple exercises after the painful stage subsides and gradually increase its duration.

Learn the correct technique of physiotherapy including exercise from a trained professional.

Avoid exercises from which you cannot recover within one hour.

Normal sexual activity can be practiced, especially when the painful stage subsides.

Avoid pregnancy during active phase of the disease.

Consult your doctor regularly for modifications in your treatment schedule depending upon your condition.

Surgery such as knee replacement if all other methods for joint mobility have failed.

therapy yourself after learning the correct technique from a qualified person.

Exercise help to relieve and prevent joint stiffness, muscle weakness, joint deformity and dependence on others. You should however avoid excessive bending of the joints. Increase the intensity and duration of the exercise gradually as you may feel tired after doing exercises to regain joint mobility and muscle strength. A simple rule is that you should recover from the 'strain' within one hour of exercises. It is important to find a correct balance between rest and exercise.

Three types of exercises help:

• those which maintain or increase joint mobility;

• those which improve muscle strength; and

• those which increase the general healthy and are beneficial to the heart and the lungs.

• *Marriage, sexual activity and motherhood.* Rheumatoid arthritis is a chronic disease which limits your ability to do normal work over a period of years. You can be sexually active although it may be difficult when you have joint pains. Although pregnancy is not contra-indicated in rheumatoid arthritis it is better to avoid pregnancy during the active phase of the disease when you require long-term medicines. Rarely the hip joint may be affected and therefore sexual activity and delivery may be difficult.

• *Regulate treatment schedule under doctor's guidance.* There is no common treatment for rheumatoid arthritis. Your doctor is likely to recommend a combination of medicines depending upon the severity of your disease, your body's acceptance of the medicines and their side-effects. Your doctor may have to modify the treatment schedule frequently in the initial stages till the correct combination and dose is achieved.

• *Surgery.* Your doctor may recommend surgery after other methods of preserving the joint and making it usable have failed. Knee joint replacement has become a very standard operation as it makes you mobile even after a prolonged illness.

Other Types of Arthritis

A group of diseases which may cause pain and swelling of the knee joint are called *arthrides*. These include:

• *Tuberculosis.* Tuberculosis commonly affects the lungs and causes cough and sputum. It may also affect the knee, especially in children. Usually only one knee is affected. Common symptoms are fever, weight loss and evidence of Tuberculosis elsewhere in the body. Your doctor is likely to recommend x-ray examination and blood tests. If these tests do not lead to confirmed diagnosis, your doctor may remove some fluid from the joint and send it for laboratory examination. It is important to detect and treat Tuberculosis of the knee at an early stage as it can damage the joint rapidly and lead to a painful, deformed knee.

• *Gout.* Gout is not a common disease. It occurs in the elderly and runs in families. In this disease excess of uric acid accumulates in the body. Symptoms develop suddenly, often overnight, with painful swelling of one or more joints with marked redness. The great toe and ankle joint are affected more than the other joints. The attack subsides on its own within a week if no treatment is taken. The second attack may occur several months or years later. However, if appropriate treatment is not taken, the attacks become more frequent, last longer and affect more joints. Gout can be precipitated by alcohol intake, heavy meal, especially meat and liver or mental stress. Your doctor will recommend a blood test for serum uric acid for making the diagnosis. Gout can be controlled with appropriate medicines.

• *Septic arthritis.* This is one of the most severe type of arthritis which occurs in children during an episode of fever. In this condition, pus collects inside the knee joints due to septic infection. This pus can damage the cartilage within a few days. Common symptoms are sudden knee pain and swelling with spiking fever in a child. The damage to the joint can be prevented by timely treatment.

Your doctor may recommend a surgical procedure to remove pus is from the joint.

ACUPUNCTURE

Causes of knee pain as per Acupuncture are the same as those detailed in the section on Allopathy. According to Acupuncture, conditions such as arthritis occur when the circulation of vital-energy and blood through special channels in the body called *acupuncture-meridians* is hindered by wind, cold, and/or dampness. Irrespective of the cause of knee pain, Acupuncture treatment opens the special channels which spread the vital energy and blood. Thus there is a long term relief from pain.

An Acupuncture practitioner will put thin stainless about one and half to two inches long steel needles at eight specific places in your leg, thigh and around the knee cap. The specific channels are opened by giving stimulation with a Chinese electro stimulator for period of twenty to thirty minutes.

Acupuncture is not a painful procedure. Once the needles are in position and the doctor starts the electrical stimulation, you will feel a very soft vibration of muscles around the place where the needle is inserted.

What is the mechanism of action of Acupuncture?

Acupuncture does not block pain. It reduces the pain by activating the release of chemical substances in the body such as *adenosine triphosphate* (which stores energy in the muscles) and *endorphins* (which are natural pain killers of the body). Thus Acupuncture relieves pain by improving the flow of vital energy and blood in the affected areas.

What are the advantages of Acupuncture?

Just like Allopathy, Acupuncture also cannot cure conditions such as osteoarthritis and rheumatoid arthritis where the damage is irreversible. The benefits of Acupuncture treatment for such cases include:

• Increased mobility and therefore more functional life-style.

• No side effects of the treatment.

- Reduced frequency of taking medicines which may have adverse side effects.

- About seventy five to eight percent relief from pain after ten to twenty treatment schedules.

- After completion of initial treatment, single booster treatment is necessary whenever pain recurs.

- Acupuncture of the ear results in weight loss of about six to eighteen kilograms over two to three months. This is because of reduced appetite and thirst, and increased volume of urine and stools.

The description of rheumatoid arthritis in Ayurvedic literature dates back to about 1000 B.C. according to Ayurveda, there are three main types of knee joint diseases:

- general;

- pain and swelling; and

- complications of some other underlying diseases. The main cause of these diseases is impaired function of the gastro-intestinal system. Decreased function of the digestive system leads to incomplete digestion and absorption of food. Some part of the partially digested food is absorbed in the body which leads to abnormalities of the blood vessels and various organs. Rheumatoid arthritis can also be the result of some diseases of the intestines.

One of the important types of inflammation of the knee joint is *Krostu shirsha*. In this condition, the *vata dosha* and blood are contaminated. The result is swelling of the knee and pain. The knee may resemble the tail of a jackal and hence the name *Krostu shirsha*.

What are the signs and symptoms of abnormalities of the knee?

According to Ayurveda, knee joint pain be similar to scorpion bite and often associated with loss of appetite, indigestion, stiffness of the body or weakness and heaviness in the left part of the chest around the heart. Some people may also complain of lack of interest in routine activities, disturbed sleep and constipation.

What is the treatment of knee pain?

Ayurveda recommends four types of treatment. These include:

- single medicines;
- simple preparations;
- compound preparations; and
- local applications.

Single medicines are prepared either from dried ginger powder to be taken with warm water or from Cassia leaves fried in ghee or mustard oil to be taken twice a day.

Simple preparations include the following:

- Decoction of equal proportion of dried ginger and stem of Heart leaved moonseed to be taken with Chebulic Myrobalan twice a day.

- Powdered seeds of Bishop's weed or Omum to be taken with warm water twice a day.

- A special decoction prepared from ten varieties of plant to be taken with castor oil every morning.

Compound preparations include Hingulesvara rasa, Maha Yogaraja guggulu, Yogaraja guggulu, Simhananda guggulu,

Visatinduka vati and Eranda paka to be taken with warm water as recommended by your doctor.

Local applications which relieve pain and swelling of the knee include:

• Fomentation with either warm sand bag or warm decoction of castor root twice a day.

• A hot paste prepared from seeds of Black phaseolus, leaves of *Rasna*, sandal, castor and Country mallow to be applied on the affected joint.

• A warm paste of wheat, castor and turmeric mixed in goat's milk or ghee to be applied on the affected part.

What are the dietary recommendations for knee pain?

Food recommended for rheumatoid arthritis include the red variety of rice, seeds of a cereal called *kodrava*, barley, dolichos bean, ginger, garlic, *patola* (a variety of small cucumber), root of pigweed, leaves of radish and fruit of bitter gourd.

HOMOEOPATHY

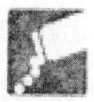

Homoeopathy also emphasizes that knee pain can be due to a wide range of causes and can occur at any age. The causes of knee joint as per the Homoeopathic system of medicine are the same as those detailed in the section on Allopathy.

What is the Homoeopathic approach to management of knee pain?

Diagnosis and correct management of knee pain as per Homoeopathy depends on the following:

Case history. A detailed case history is the foundation of Homoeopathic treatment. Your doctor will ask you to describe

• symptoms such as the exact location of the pain, factors which increase or decrease it and any other associated symptoms;

• onset of the disease such as injury;

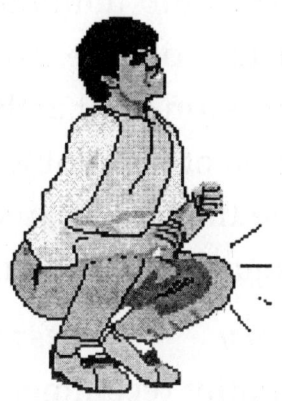

• family history. According to Homoeopathy, osteoarthritis is more common among those who have family history of diabetes.

General Examination. Your doctor will examine you in detail before establishing the diagnosis. Skin injuries and dryness of skin may be due to some auto-immune disease. Deformities of the joint may indicate rheumatoid arthritis and examination of the joint will help to determine the likely cause of pain such as injury or infection.

Laboratory investigations. Homoeopathy recommends x-rays and some blood tests not only to establish a diagnosis but also to assess the progress of the disease. Commonly recommended blood tests are haemoglobin (Hb) blood cell counts, erythrocyte sedimentation rate (ESR), Serum Uric Acid and R. A. Factor.

What is the aim of Homoeopathic treatment for knee pain?

Homoeopathy offers a wide range of remedies which often cure or at least reduce the pain through:

• **Constitutional treatment.** These are medicines which are prescribed on the basis of detailed individual case history. These medicines act on your defence mechanism by modifying the abnormal immune response and restoring the balance of the immune system.

• **Miasmatic treatment.** Some diseases which can cause knee pain may run in families. This is because of inherited characteristics which increase susceptibility to diseases. Homoeopathic medicines eradicate these inherited and harmful characteristics and thus allow cure of the disease by appropriate medicines. For example, *Tuberculinum* is prescribed for those with family history of Tuberculosis and Thuja and Medorrhinum for those with family history of arthritis or diabetes.

- **Specific treatment.** Homoeopathy recommends specific medicines in case of acute pain or when there is advanced, irreversible damage to the joint. These medicines have a direct action on the joint, reduce pain, relieve the muscle spasm, repair muscle wasting, discourage the formation of adhesions and therefore enhances mobility of the joint. Constitutional treatment is prescribed only after acute pain subsides.

What is the management of knee pain?

Homoeopathy recommends general management as well as specific treatment for various causes of knee pain.

Medical management of knee pain. Homoeopathic medicines are very effective for treatment of knee pain. When the diseases is very advanced and the joint deformity is severe and irreversible, surgery is essential. However, even at this stage Homoeopathic medicines help to relieve pain and maintain some mobility.

There are several Homoeopathic medicines to treat knee pain. Some of these are Rhus Tox; Bryonea; Gaultheria; Viscum Album; Calcium Salts; Lithium Carb and Strontium Carb. Your Homoeopath is the best person to decide the medicine and its dose depending upon your condition. *It is important to remember that Homoeopathic medicines are very effective if treatment is started early.* Detailed below is the treatment of specific causes of knee pain.

- **Osteoarthritis.** Homoeopathy recommends medicines which have specific effect on specific joints. The aim of the treatment is to lessen the pain, reduce stiffness and provide comfort. O.A. Nosode is a medicine prepared from disease tissues of a person suffering from osteoarthritis which has been used successfully in treatment of knee pain due to osteoarthritis. Regular treatment with this medicine slows the progress of destructive process as can be seen through repeated x-rays. The severity of the symptoms also decrease.

- **Autoimmune diseases.** Autoimmune diseases which cause knee pain such as rheumatoid Arthritis can be managed effectively with Homoeopathic medicines. This is because these medicines stimulates natural defence mechanism of the body and helps it to function at an optimum level. Homoeopathy recommends *constitutional medicines* which are selected on the basis of case history and not just the local symptoms. These medicines not only relieve the pain, but also build your vitality to a level where you can fight the disease.

- **Injury to the knee or surrounding tissue.** Arnica, a Homoeopathic medicine is very effective in injuries such as sprains

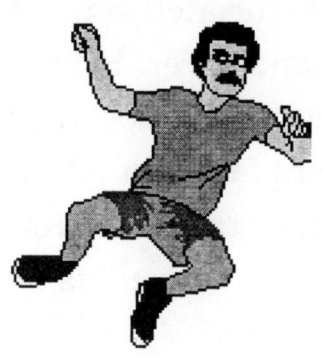

and ligament tears. It reduces the pain and initiates and accelerates the healing process.

- **Septic arthritis.** Many people believe that Homoeopathy is not effective in acute infections as it acts slowly. This is not true. There are several Homoeopathic medicines which cure infection and reduce associated symptoms such as pain and fever. However, your Homoeopath may recommend treatment by an Orthopaedic surgeon if the infection is very acute or there is risk of complications.

- **Gout.** Homoeopathic medicines reduce serum uric levels and improve the body's normal constitution.

Homoeopathy also recommends physiotherapy to improve joint mobility and enhance the effect of the medicines.

General management of knee pain. Homoeopathy also recommends general management of knee pain with a well balanced diet, preventing obesity and regular exercise as recommended by a physiotherapist.

What are the strengths of Homoeopathic medicines?

The main advantages of Homoeopathic treatment for knee joint pain include its ability to:

• Provide maximum comfort and mobility with minimum disability.

• Prevent deformities.

• Slow down and occasionally reverse the degenerative process.

• Repair the damaged joint tissues.

• Prevent further complications.

In addition, Homoeopathic medicines do not have any side-effects.

What are the limitations of Homoeopathy?

Homoeopathic medicines are not very effective in advanced cases and hence your Homoeopath may recommend treatment by an orthopaedic surgeon. He/she may also recommend pain killers such as Paracetamol if the pain is severe and the mobility is greatly limited.

NATURE CURE

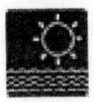

Causes of knee pain as per Nature Cure are the same as those described in the section on Allopathy.

What is the treatment of keen pain?

Nature Cure recommends the following pain relief formula:

R — Rest and Relaxation

I — Ice Application

C — Cold Compress

E — Elevation

Other treatment options recommended by Nature Cure to reduce knee pain include:

• *Knee joint pack.* Apply a cold cloth, a dry cloth and a blanket in the same order around the joint. The size of the cloth and blanket should be the same as the size of the knee. Keep this pack for one hour every night.

• *Ice massage.* Rub ice cubes over and around the knee joint till the skin becomes red and there is a numb sensation. Next, apply several layers of dry cloth on the knee till it becomes warm.

• *Fomentation.* Keep a hot water bottle or sand bag till the knee joint becomes as warm as you can tolerate. Immediately apply cold cloth on the knee and cover it with flannel for one hour.

• *Hot and cold applications.* You can do this either with stream of water or cloth. Pour the hot water or apply a cloth dipped in hot water for two minutes on the knee. Immediately pour chilled water or apply a cloth dipped in chilled water for thirty seconds. Repeat this process four to five times. Hot and cold applications are recommended three times a week.

• *Mud application.* Collect clean black mud and remove stones and other impurities. Soak this mud in a pot for twenty four hours and make a paste. Apply this paste on the knee joint and allow it to become dry and wash it with cold water. Dry the knee quickly. It is better to apply the mud in sun-shine.

• *Massage.* Oil massage to the knee can relieve pain. You should however learn the correct technique of oil massage from a Nature Cure practitioner.

• *Red coloured rays.* Apply the red colour rays from sun-light using red coloured glass for fifteen minutes.

The treatment options detailed above improve blood circulation of the knee, relieving congestion and remove "poisons". The pain and swelling therefore reduces.

Exercise. Regular exercise prevents pain due to stiffness of the muscles around the joints. Walking is a good exercise. If walking is painful, stretch your knees and move them sideways to improve muscle tone and blood circulation.

Diet. Eat a diet consisting of vegetables especially potatoes, salads, fruits, juices, soups, unpolished rice, wheat germ and whole wheat bread. It is better to limit protein intake. You should therefore avoid meat, cheese, milk, milk products peas and beans. You should also avoid fried foods, white refined flour, sugar and excessive salt. Potatoes can be taken specially as vegetable.

Fasting. Your Nature Cure practitioner may suggest fast for three to seven days. You can take fruit juices of lemon, grape fruit and orange during the fast.

Herbal remedies. Nature Cure recommends the following three herbal remedies for relief of knee pain:

1. Raw potato juice is a highly alkaline and is very effective for gout. It reduces uric acid level in the blood. You should take a few ounces of potato juice everyday before break fast. If you do not like the taste or find it difficult to extract the juice, dilute it in warm water.

2. Chew and eat two to three juniper berries one hour before lunch. Swallow two to four mustard seeds after lunch. During the day drink only the water in which potatoes were boiled.

3. Drink parsley tea.

UNANI

The Unani system of medicine is based on *humoural* theory of Hippocrates: blood, phlegm, bile and black bile. These *humours* are defined as moist and fluid substance produced in the liver from the food ingested and are capable of carrying nutrients to the body. The contamination of *humours* is said to take place if they are not prepared in the liver and are not able to transport nutrients to the body. The body is healthy when these four humours remain intermixed in the blood in a specific balance. Various body fluids including the synovial fluid in the joints are derived out of these four humours in a specific proportion.

According to Unani system of medicine, the joints pain or *Wajaul Mafasil* is the result of abnormalities in the normal balance of the four *humours* in the synovial fluids. The result is derangement of *temperament* of the joints, absorption of these abnormal *humours* in various organs where they either stagnate or stagnate. This abnormality is more when the causative factor foul bodies which disrupts the digestive process. As a result, blood gets contaminated with some abnormal "matter". There are four types of knee pain depending upon the type of abnormal *humour:*

1. Damavi;

2. Valghami;

3. Saudavi; and

4. Safravi.

What are the signs and symptoms of various types of knee pain?

In 'Damvi' type of knee pain, there is excessive redness of the skin over the joints with sever pain and swelling. In 'Safravi type there is slight yellow discolouration of the skin around the joints. The swelling is less marked but the skin over the joint is warm and itchy. Pain is also present. 'Balghami' type is recognised by soft swelling; sever pain and the

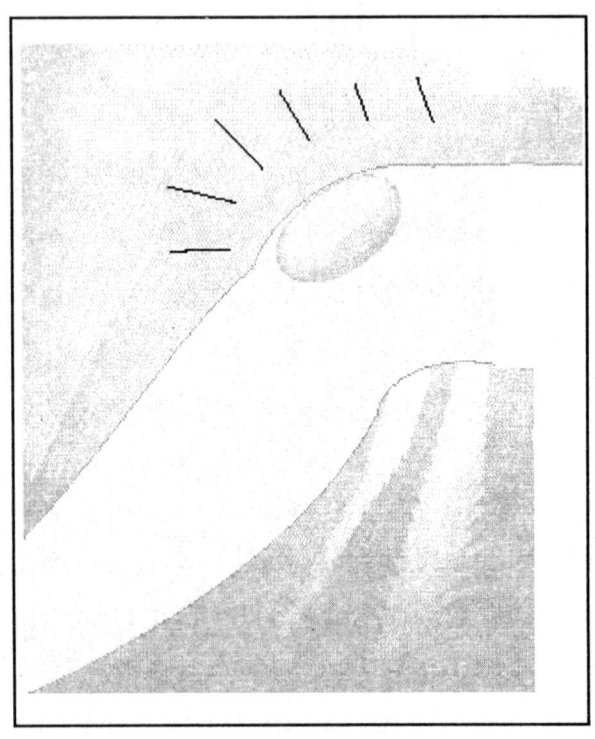

joint is painful to touch. The area around the joint is also slightly painful. The skin on the joints in 'Saudavi' type is either black or blue with hard swelling.

What is the treatment of knee pain?

The Unani system of medicine recommends three types of treatment for knee pain. These are:

(1) single medicines;

(2) local applications; and

(3) regimental therapy.

Single medicines are prepared from any one of the following plants: Sweet Colchicum, Betel nut, Opium, Violet, Marsh Mallow, Cirata, Tamarind, Prunes, Large

Raisin, Indian Laburnum, Chamomile, Crecent beans, Colocynth, Orchids, Dill fruit, Aloe, Myrrh, Fenugreek, Linseed, Vitex, and Turmeric.

Single medicines are prescribed in various combination and dose ranging from new milligrams six grams according depending upon the condition of the disease. None of the above medicines have any known adverse effects.

Local applications can be done with any one of the following:

Castor oil, Chamomile oil, Spikenard, Costus oil, Almond oil, Wax oil, Kitchen fat, Goat fat and Balsam oil.

Regimental therapy includes the following:

1. Application of warm compress of decoction prepared mainly from neem, mint, chamomile, cresent beans and fenugreek on the affected joints.

2. Medicated bath in which the affected joints are immersed in luke warm decoction prepared as for warm compress.

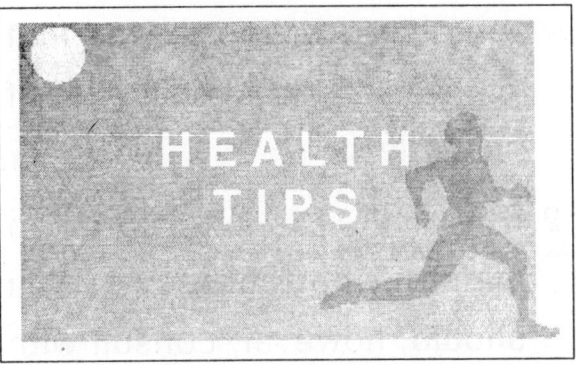

HEALTH TIPS

1. Pain-killers may relieve pain temporarily but in the long run they just cover the symptoms while the disease progresses further. They also inhibit the production of a compound that occurs naturally in the cartilage cushioning the joints. It is,

therefore, recommended that you avoid indiscriminate use of pain-killers.

2. Exercise is important to maintain normal health. You should, however, consult with your doctor before starting strenuous exercises.

3. Cupping, which is a minor surgical procedure in which the abnormal fluid or matter is removed from the joint.

Definitions

Adenosine triphosphate is a chemical compound which serves to store energy in the muscles.

Arthroscope is a special tube like instrument used for arthroscopy.

Arthroscopy is the examination of the interior of a joint performed by inserting a specially designed tube through a small incision. It is usually performed on the knee joint for (1) biopsy; (2) diagnosis; or (3) removal of loose bodies in the joint space.

Capsule is a well defined structure of the body which encloses an organ or a part of the body.

Cartilage is a type of supportive tissue found mainly in the joints and various rigid tubes such as the wind pipe, nose and ear. It does not contain any blood vessels.

Endorphins are chemical substances secreted in a part of the brain. These are natural pain killers.

Hamstrings are a group of three muscles in the back of the thigh.

High tibial osteotomy is a surgical procedure in which the damaged or deformed upper end of the leg bone is removed.

Ligaments are white shiny, flexible bands of tissue which bind joints and connect various bones and cartilages.

Meniscus is a curved cartilage in the knee and other joints. In the knee they are shaped like a half-moon.

Pseudogout is an arthritic disease in which calcium deposits are found in some joints. It is found in people above fifty years of age who have osteoarthritis and diabetes mellitus.

Quadriceps is composed of four muscles which form the large dense mass on the front and sides of the thigh. The four muscles unite in at the lower part of the thigh to form a tendon which is attached to the knee cap.

Synovial fluid is a transparent liquid which resembles the white of an egg which acts as a lubricating agent for many joints and tendons.

Tendons are white glistening bands of tissue which attach muscle to the bones. They are extremely strong and flexible and inelastic.

References

Allopathy

Goldberg VM, Ketteldamp DB, Colyer RA: Osteoarthritis of the knee. Osteoarthritis: Diagnosis and Medical/Surgical Management; Edited by RW Moskowitz, DS Howell, VM Goldberg, Philadelphia, World Bank Saunders, 1992.

McAlindon T, Dieppe PARTICIPANTS: The medical management of osteoarthritis of the knee: an inflammatory issue? British Journal of Rheumatology, 29:471-473, 1990.

Scott JC, Hochberg MC: Arthritic and other musculoskeletal diseases. Chronic Disease Epidemiology and Control; Edited by RC Browson, PL Remington, JR Davis, Washington DC, American Public Health Association, 1993.

Acupuncture

"Electro-myographic-study of Acupuncture Therapy for knee-pain", British Journal of Acupuncture Vol. Ii No. 1 - 1988

"34-cases of Effusion of knee-treated by Acupuncture", British Journal of Acupuncture Vol.; 14 no. 2 Page 47

Mori H., Modern Acupuncture

Ayurveda

Astanga Hridaya Samhita

Bhaisajyaratnavali

Cakradatta

Caraka Samhita

Susru ta Samhita

Nature Cure

Walker Norman, Fresh Vegetable
and Fruit Juice.

Vogel A., Swiss Nature Doctor